CANCER-FIGHTING CUISINE

NUTRIENT-PACKED RECIPES AND GUIDANCE FOR EVERY STAGE OF CHEMOTHERAPY

JOY DANIELS

Copyright © 2023 by Joy Daniel

TABLE OF CONTENT

INTRODUCTION 5

CHAPTER 1: UNDERSTANDING THE CONNECTION 8

- The relationship between nutrition and cancer. 10

- The role of a balanced diet in cancer treatment 14

- How chemotherapy affects the body's nutritional needs...18

CHAPTER 2: BUILDING YOUR NUTRITIONAL FOUNDATION 23

- Navigating dietary guidelines before, during, and after chemotherapy.................................25

- Essential nutrients for supporting the immune system and overall health 29

- Customizing your meal plan based on individual needs and preferences 33

CHAPTER 3: COOKING FOR COMFORT AND HEALING 37

- Recipes tailored for managing chemotherapy side effects...39

- Delicious and nourishing dishes to soothe the palate 47

- Easy-to-follow meal preparation tips and techniques 54

CHAPTER 4: NUTRIENT-PACKED RECIPE COLLECTION 62

- A diverse array of recipes featuring cancer-fighting ingredients 64

- Culinary inspiration for every stage of chemotherapy 75

CHAPTER 5: SUSTAINING WELLNESS BEYOND TREATMENT 80

- Strategies for transitioning to a post-chemotherapy diet 83

- Long-term dietary recommendations for cancer survivors 88

- A roadmap for maintaining a health-conscious lifestyle after treatment 94

CONCLUSION 100

INTRODUCTION

In the fight against cancer, nutrition is essential for maintaining the body's fortitude and vigor. Introducing "Cancer-Fighting Cuisine: Nutrient-Packed Recipes and Guidance for Every Stage of Chemotherapy," an extensive cookbook created with skill, kindness, and knowledge. You will travel on a transforming journey via these pages, where you will find a plethora of healthy recipes and priceless nutritional advice designed especially for cancer patients.

This book is more than just a compilation of recipes; it is a source of inspiration and evidence of the need to provide physical and emotional support to oneself when facing adversity. This comprehensive guide smoothly blends delicious flavors with the therapeutic benefits of carefully chosen components, drawing on the most recent research as well as the experience of seasoned cancer nutritionists. Every recipe is painstakingly created to supply vital nutrients, support your immune system, and lessen typical side effects of chemotherapy, whether you're looking for solace in tried-and-true favorites or exploring novel foods to pique your curiosity.

However, Cancer-Fighting Cuisine isn't just for cooking. It gives you a thorough grasp of how important diet is to your recovery process. You'll receive professional advice on meal planning, dietary requirements, and useful strategies for handling nutritional difficulties, giving you the information and self-assurance you need to make decisions that are best for your health. This book gives you the tools to take control of your health and make sure that you not only survive but thrive during your chemotherapy journey. It is empowering and uplifting.

Get ready to go on a life-changing gastronomic journey that will nourish your body, boost your spirits, and give you the energy to greet every day with renewed vigor. As you peruse the pages of "Cancer-Fighting Cuisine," allow the perfume of healthful foods and the promise of healing to uplift you. Together, we'll set off on a voyage of resiliency, rejuvenation, and delectable exploration, demonstrating that the power of wholesome, thoughtfully prepared meals can illuminate the path toward wellness and hope even in the face of adversity.

CHAPTER 1:
UNDERSTANDING THE CONNECTION

The complex and frequently disregarded relationship between cancer and nutrition is a significant element of the whole picture of human health. This is the insightful chapter "Understanding the Connection between Cancer and Nutrition." Welcome. In these pages, we will dig into the complex world of molecular biology and examine how our diets can influence the course of one of the greatest threats to humankind: cancer.

The word "cancer," which conjures up feelings of dread and anxiety, refers to a broad range of illnesses rather than just one. But among all of this intricacy, there is one astounding fact to be aware of: the decisions we make about our daily nutrition can affect how well our bodies fight this powerful enemy. This chapter takes us on an intriguing voyage to decipher the complex scientific theories underlying the connection between diet and cancer.

We will explore the maze of cellular biology and learn how some foods can serve as protectors, enhancing our defenses against disease and strengthening our cells from the inside out. Together, we will investigate cutting-edge research that highlights the critical role that a balanced diet plays in both prevention and as an essential element of comprehensive cancer care.

We will explore the cultural and historical backgrounds that have influenced our understanding of food and its therapeutic qualities in addition to the scientific domain. We will explore the ageless knowledge that emphasizes the significance of nutrition in the face of illness, from traditional medical practices to contemporary advances in oncology.

Get ready to be enthralled by the inspirational tales, scientific discoveries, and wisdom that will be revealed in the pages to follow. You will acquire priceless knowledge as we explore the complexities of the relationship between diet and cancer. This knowledge will enable you to make wise decisions and will give you hope and control when faced with hardship.

Accept this chapter as a guiding light that will help you comprehend the significant influence that your dietary decisions can have on your path to wellness. Let's set off on a transformative journey together, bridging the science-food gap and shedding light on the way to a healthier, cancer-fighting future.

- The relationship between nutrition and cancer

1. **Cancer Prevention**: Phytochemicals and Antioxidants: Various phytochemicals present in fruits, vegetables, and whole grains, as well as

nutrients like vitamins C and E, function as antioxidants. They lower the chance of cellular damage and mutation by eliminating dangerous free radicals from the body.

Fiber and Digestive Health: Eating meals high in fiber promotes good digestion and weight maintenance. Furthermore, a healthy digestive system lowers the risk of colorectal cancer by limiting the exposure of colon cells to possible carcinogens.

Balanced Fats: Reducing saturated fat intake and consuming omega-3 fatty acids, which are present in walnuts, flaxseeds, and fish, can help control inflammation in the body, which has been connected to the development of cancer.

2. **Cancer Progression and Treatment**: Immune **System Support**: A healthy diet makes the immune system stronger, which improves its ability to recognize and eliminate cancer cells. The immune system is heavily dependent on

several nutrients, including zinc, selenium, and vitamins A, D, and E.

Sustaining a Healthy Body Weight: Numerous cancer kinds are significantly increased by obesity. A healthy diet and regular exercise help control weight, lower the risk of cancer, and promote general health both during and after treatment.

Handling Side Effects of Treatment: The side effects of radiation and chemotherapy can be lessened by eating specific foods and nutrients. For instance, diets high in protein promote tissue healing following treatments, and ginger relieves nausea.

3. **Changing the Expression of Genes**: Epigenetics Gene expression can be influenced by nutrients via epigenetic processes. Certain food ingredients can alter gene activity without altering the underlying DNA sequence. Understanding how dietary decisions can affect

cancer risk and progression is a promising area of research.

4. **Particular Nutrients and Their Functions**:

Vitamin D: Studies indicate that having enough vitamin D in the body may reduce the risk of developing several malignancies, such as colon, prostate, and breast cancer. It helps maintain the immune system and controls the proliferation of cells.

Cruciferous Vegetables: Broccoli, cauliflower, and Brussels sprouts are examples of vegetables that include substances that have been connected to a lower risk of cancer. Certain substances, like sulforaphane, have been demonstrated to stop cancer cells from proliferating.

Turmeric and Curcumin: The active component of turmeric, curcumin, has antioxidant and anti-inflammatory qualities and may inhibit the growth and survival of cancer cells.

Comprehending the subtleties of these associations enables individuals to make knowledgeable dietary decisions that can reduce the risk of cancer, support cancer therapy, and improve general health. This information provides a ray of hope as research into the intricate relationship between nutrition and cancer continues, showing the real benefits of a thoughtful, balanced diet on cancer prevention, treatment outcomes, and survivability.

- The role of a balanced diet in cancer treatment

1. **Foods High in Protein**:

Ingredients: Fish, eggs, poultry, lean meats, lentils, tofu, and nuts.

Function: During cancer treatment, proteins are necessary for immune system support, tissue repair, and muscle mass maintenance.

Recipe ideas include baked salmon, grilled chicken breast, lentil soup, whole-grain toast with almond butter, or a smoothie made with fruits, Greek yoghurt, and spinach.

2. **Whole Grains**: **Ingredients:** pasta made from whole grains, barley, quinoa, whole wheat, and oats.

Function: Fiber, vitamins, and minerals are provided by whole grains. They facilitate regular energy release and aid in digestive regulation.

Preparation options include brown rice stir-fried with tofu and vegetables, quinoa salad with vegetables, and whole-grain spaghetti with roasted veggies.

3. **Fruits and Vegetables**: Components include carrots, colored bell peppers, cruciferous

vegetables (broccoli, kale, Brussels sprouts), citrus fruits, berries, and leafy greens.

Role: Packed with fiber, vitamins, and antioxidants, fruits and vegetables boost immunity and lower inflammation.

Preparation options include stir-fried broccoli and bell peppers, roasted vegetable medley, smoothies made with spinach and berries, and fresh fruit salads.

4. **Good Fats:**

Ingredients: avocado, olive oil, walnuts, almonds, chia seeds, flaxseeds, and fatty fish (mackerel, salmon).

Role: Good fats enhance general health by promoting energy, assisting in the absorption of nutrients, and having anti-inflammatory qualities.

Preparation options include chia seed pudding, salmon salad with olive oil dressing, avocado toast, and a snack of mixed nuts and seeds.

5. **Hydration:**

Ingredients: Water; herbal teas; fruit- and herb-infused water.

Role: Hydration is key to controlling adverse symptoms such as tiredness, nausea, and dry mouth. Drinking enough water promotes all body processes and aids in the removal of pollutants.

Preparation options include ginger tea, cucumber-mint-infused water, or just plain water with a wedge of lemon.

6. **Herbs and Spices:**

Ingredients: mint, cinnamon, ginger, garlic, and turmeric.

Role: Some herbs and spices have antioxidant and anti-inflammatory qualities that help boost the immune system and manage the side effects of treatment.

Preparation: Roasted veggies with garlic and herbs, hot water infused with ginger, or a cool drink with mint and lemon.

Cancer patients can assist their bodies throughout treatment by adding these components to well-balanced meals. A trained dietitian or healthcare professional can also assist in customizing a nutrition plan to meet the needs and tastes of each individual, making sure that the diet meets the particular requirements of the cancer treatment plan.

- *How chemotherapy affects the body's nutritional needs*

Chemotherapy is a potent and frequently life-saving cancer treatment that can have a major impact on the body's dietary requirements. Patients and healthcare professionals need to be aware of these changes to create a customized nutrition plan that promotes general health and helps with treatment-related side effects management. This is a detailed investigation into the impact of chemotherapy on the body's dietary requirements:

1. **Increased Energy and Protein Requirements:** The body may require more protein and energy during chemotherapy. To maintain muscle mass, assist tissue healing, and maintain energy levels, the body needs more calories and protein.

Chemotherapy patients frequently experience exhaustion, weight loss, and muscle atrophy; therefore, it's critical to eat enough protein and calories to avoid malnutrition.

2. **Difficulties with the Digestive System:** Chemotherapy can harm the lining of the digestive tract, resulting in problems like vomiting, diarrhea, mouth sores, and nausea.

The capacity to eat, digest, and absorb nutrients may be hampered by these symptoms.

It might be difficult to maintain a balanced diet when taking certain chemotherapy medicines since they alter taste buds and cause changes in food aversions and preferences.

3. **Nutrient Absorption and Metabolism:** Chemotherapy may impede the body's gastrointestinal tract's capacity to absorb nutrients, including vitamins and minerals. Nutritional deficits may result from this malabsorption.

Certain chemotherapy medications may affect the metabolism of the body, changing how nutrients are used and stored. This may have an impact on overall nutritional status and weight management.

4. **Immune System Suppression:** Immune system suppression brought on by chemotherapy increases a patient's susceptibility to infections.

To maintain immune function and aid the body in fending off infections and recovering from therapies, proper nutrition is essential.

Sufficient consumption of vitamins, minerals, and antioxidants becomes essential for enhancing the immune system and lowering the chance of infection.

5. **Hydration and Electrolyte Balance:** Dehydration and electrolyte abnormalities can result from chemotherapy-induced vomiting, diarrhea, and increased urination. For optimal organ function and general health, electrolyte balance and appropriate hydration must be maintained.

To treat severe dehydration and electrolyte imbalances brought on by chemotherapy side effects, intravenous fluids and electrolyte supplements could be required.

6. **Psychological and Emotional Factors:** Cancer diagnosis and treatment are frequently

accompanied by psychological stress, worry, and sadness. Appetite and food decisions are significantly influenced by emotional health.

Patients who need assistance managing emotional pressures and maintaining a positive relationship with food can benefit from supportive interventions, psychotherapy, and mindfulness techniques.

Comprehending these obstacles enables medical professionals to create customized dietary regimens tailored to the unique requirements of patients receiving chemotherapy. To make sure patients get enough nutrients, control treatment-related side effects, and enhance overall quality of life both during and after chemotherapy, these regimens may involve dietary adjustments, nutritional supplements, and supportive therapies.

CHAPTER 2: BUILDING YOUR NUTRITIONAL FOUNDATION

Building a solid nutritional foundation is like building a strong fortress in the complex maze of cancer therapy. Greetings and welcome to the insightful chapter "Building Your Nutritional Foundation," where we will take a revolutionary trip into the core of nutrition. You will learn the value of a well-balanced diet here, in the middle of the flurry of emotions and the disorder of treatments—a fundamental component that may support your resilience, give you confidence, and open the door to recovery.

Think of your body as an exquisite, detailed, and breathtaking temple. Similar to how a temple needs a strong base to endure over time, your body too needs a strong dietary foundation to tolerate the rigors of cancer therapy. This chapter reveals the methods for building this foundation, including the essential nutrients, dietary recommendations, and customized meal plans that will strengthen your body, uplift your spirit, and accelerate your recuperation.

We will explore the maze of food options together, learning about the roles that lipids, proteins, carbs, vitamins, and minerals play in the complex dance of cellular renewal. By customizing each suggestion to your particular requirements and interests, we will help you understand the mystery around calorie counts and portion sizes. Whether you're looking for the comforting embrace of comfort food or the energizing zest of colorful, nutrient-dense meals, this chapter will walk you through the process of becoming a more fed, balanced, and bright version of yourself.

You will find not just dietary guidance in the pages that follow, but also a recipe for strength, a resilience map, and a road map for revitalization. You will discover the methods to turn ordinary meals into powerful elixirs that are packed with the restorative energy your body longs for as we unravel the secrets of creating your nutritional foundation.

Get ready to go on an in-depth journey where food becomes more than just a source of nutrition; it becomes an ally, a comfort, and a source of power. Allow this chapter to serve as your beacon of light, showing you the way to a happier, healthier version of yourself. Together, we will build a nutritious foundation that will support you toward a future of hope and wellness while being steadfast and unwavering in the face of hardship.

- Navigating dietary guidelines before, during, and after chemotherapy

1. **Before Chemotherapy:** It is important to focus on a balanced and nutrient-rich diet to prepare the body for chemotherapy. To better withstand the impending therapies, this phase seeks to

strengthen the body's immune system and general health.

Increased Protein Consumption: To develop and repair tissues, eat lean meats, poultry, fish, dairy products, legumes, and nuts. For instance, grilled salmon offers high-quality protein and omega-3 fatty acids.

Foods High in Antioxidants: Include vibrant fruits and vegetables such as carrots, spinach, and berries. They supply antioxidants and vitamins. A spinach and berry smoothie is a fantastic option.

Hydration: To stay hydrated, consume a lot of water, herbal teas, and clear soups. For a cool twist, add cucumber and mint slices to the water.

2. **Throughout Chemotherapy:** The body experiences a great deal of stress throughout chemotherapy. Enough nutrition boosts the immune system, promotes healing, and helps control the negative effects of treatment.

Soft, Easy-to-Digest Foods: Go for foods like yoghurt, boiled potatoes, and plain rice that are easy on the stomach. Steer clear of oily and spicy foods. A straightforward rice porridge topped with sautéed veggies is both nourishing and cozy.

Ginger provides anti-nausea qualities that help with nausea management. Nausea can be reduced with ginger tea or water infused with ginger. Toast or simple crackers are gentle on the stomach.

Small, Frequent Meals: Spread out your nutrient-dense meals throughout the day rather than consuming huge ones. Eat some yoghurt, almonds, or whole-grain crackers as a snack.

3. **Following Chemotherapy:** The body must heal and regenerate following chemotherapy. Foods high in nutrients promote healing, increase vitality, and improve general health.

Protein for Recovery: Keep highlighting foods high in protein to support muscular growth and tissue repair. Lentil soup and grilled chicken breast are great sources of protein.

Whole Grains & Fiber: Whole grains offer long-lasting energy. Examples of these are brown rice, quinoa, and oats. Foods high in fibre, such as whole grains, fruits, and vegetables, improve digestion and fend off constipation.

Bone Health: Consume dairy products, leafy greens, almonds, and fortified plant-based milk to enhance your diet's calcium and vitamin D content. A salad with spinach and almonds is nourishing and tasty.

Savor every piece of food while concentrating on eating mindfully. To guarantee a well-rounded nutrient intake, eat a range of foods.

To follow these dietary recommendations, meals must be modified to accommodate each person's tolerances and tastes. Making use of the individualized advice provided by a registered dietitian with expertise in oncology nutrition helps guarantee that the diet best supports the body before, during, and following chemotherapy.

- Essential nutrients for supporting the immune system and overall health

1. **Vitamin C:**

Function: Vitamin C, which is well-known for its antioxidant qualities, strengthens the immune system by promoting the development and functionality of white blood cells.

Citrus fruits (lemons and oranges), strawberries, bell peppers, broccoli, and kiwis are some of the sources. For instance, a tasty and vitamin C-rich dish is a crisp citrus salad with bell peppers and strawberries.

2. **Vitamin D:**

Purpose: Immune system performance and the body's defense against infections depend on vitamin D. It affects bone health as well.

Sources: Sunlight exposure, egg yolks, fortified dairy or plant-based milk, fatty fish (salmon, mackerel). A boiled egg, a side of sautéed spinach, and grilled salmon make for a wholesome, high-vitamin D lunch.

3. **Zinc:** Zinc has a crucial role in immune cell formation and function, promoting wound healing and lowering inflammation.

Sources: Whole grains, nuts (almonds and cashews), poultry, beef, and beans. Along with other vital elements, a hearty stir-fried dish of beef and vegetables with brown rice contains zinc.

4. **Probiotics:** Function: Probiotics are good bacteria that enhance gut health and have an impact on immunological responses and general health.

Sources: Fermented foods such as kimchi, sauerkraut, kefir, and yoghurt. A delicious approach to including probiotics in the diet is to make a parfait for breakfast consisting of yoghurt, granola, and mixed berries.

5. **Omega-3 Fatty Acids:**

Function: Due to its anti-inflammatory qualities, omega-3 fatty acids promote cardiovascular and immune system health.

Sources: Walnuts, flaxseeds, chia seeds, and fatty fish (sardines, salmon). Flaxseed dressing on a salmon and avocado wrap delivers taste and omega-3 fatty acids.

6. **Iron:**

Function: Iron is necessary for the body to produce red blood cells, which carry oxygen throughout the body and maintain the immune system and general vigor.

Red meat, chicken, fish, lentils, spinach, and fortified cereals are some of the sources. A balanced, high-iron lunch can be had with a side of grilled chicken and a substantial lentil soup with spinach.

7. **Antioxidants (Vitamin E, Selenium):** **Function:** Antioxidants help the immune system fight off infections and shield cells from harm.

Sources: Whole grains, spinach, broccoli, and nuts (almonds, sunflower seeds). Antioxidants and other vital elements can be found in a nutrient-dense salad made with spinach, mixed nuts, and a drizzle of olive oil.

Including these nutrients in a varied, well-balanced diet helps to support general health and a strong immune system. People can make tasty, fulfilling meals that boost their body's natural defensive mechanisms and improve their general well-being by combining different food sources.

- Customizing your meal plan based on individual needs and preferences

Making a meal plan unique to each person's requirements and tastes is crucial to developing a fun and long-lasting approach to nutrition. Customizing a meal plan to an individual's specific nutritional needs, preferences, and objectives can improve adherence and general health. This is a thorough explanation of how to alter a meal plan, along with pertinent examples:

1. **Being Aware of Dietary Restrictions:** For instance, if a person is lactose intolerant, they can choose plant-based substitutes like soy or almond milk or lactose-free dairy products.

2. **Taking Allergies Into Account:** For instance, meals can be made without nuts for a person who is allergic to them, or they can use substitutes like seeds (like sunflower seeds) for extra texture and nutrients.

33 |CANCER-FIGHTING CUISINE

3. **Balancing Macronutrients:** For instance, people who want to lose weight can concentrate on consuming more fiber and protein. Quinoa, grilled chicken breast, and an assortment of vegetables may make for a satisfying and nutrient-dense meal.

4. **Adapting for Health Conditions:** For instance, people with diabetes might concentrate on controlling their intake of carbohydrates. Lean protein (chicken or tofu), non-starchy veggies, and a tiny amount of whole carbohydrates (quinoa or brown rice) can all be found in a balanced meal.

5. **Including Personal Preferences:** For instance, a person with a love for Mediterranean food may design a menu that includes grilled fish, olives, whole-grain couscous, and an assortment of vibrant veggies.

6. **Taking into Account Cultural and Ethical Decisions:** For instance, vegans and vegetarians

can add plant-based protein sources like beans, lentils, tofu, and a range of vegetables to their meal plans. A tasty and filling vegan option is a stir-fry with tofu, broccoli, and bell peppers over brown rice.

7. **Portion Control and Mindful Eating:** As an illustration, those who are trying to control their portions can visually deceive their minds into thinking they are getting by with lower portions by using smaller plates and bowls. This can be combined with mindful eating practices to improve the whole eating experience.

8. **Adaptable Meal Schedule:**

Example: While some people choose to eat three larger meals a day, others may choose smaller, more frequent meals throughout the day. Adapting the timing of meals to individual schedules and dietary requirements can improve plan adherence.

9. **Trying Out Different Cooking Methods:**

Example: You may make delicious dishes with common ingredients by roasting, grilling, steaming, or sautéing them to suit a variety of palates. For instance, roasted veggies with a balsamic glaze can enhance the flavor and depth of a dish.

Not only can a customized meal plan fulfil dietary requirements, but it can also enhance and satisfy the eating experience. A customized meal plan can be developed by taking into account each person's needs, preferences, and objectives. This guarantees that the food is not only nourishing but also enjoyable and fulfilling in day-to-day living.

CHAPTER 3: COOKING FOR COMFORT AND HEALING

Every kitchen has a sanctuary at its center, where comforting fragrances waft through the air and ingredients combine to create elixirs of healing. Welcome to the magical chapter "Cooking for Comfort and Healing," where delicate caregiving blends with culinary expertise. Here, amid the sounds of pans sizzling and spices wafting, you'll set off on a journey that goes beyond simple sustenance to replenish the soul.

When things are tough and you feel vulnerable, there is great comfort in cooking. It's a ritual, an intimate dance between the hands that prepare and the hearts that seek comfort, rather than just a simple melding of flavors' and textures. This chapter honors the ability of food to serve as more than just a source of nourishment; it may also act as a source of warmth, a spiritual healer, and a ray of hope.

Imagine the rich aroma of a pot of soup simmering on the stove or the soft kneading of bread by skilled hands. These are not only culinary pursuits; they are acts of love, infused with the deep knowledge that feeding transcends the material world. It reaches the very center of who we are, providing nourishment for both our tired bodies and souls.

You will find a plethora of recipes in the pages that follow, all of which have been painstakingly prepared and selected for their capacity to soothe and heal. Every meal is a testament to the soothing power of mindful cooking, from delicately flavored teas that calm the senses to velvety soups that embrace like a warm embrace. You will learn from these recipes that the kitchen can serve as a haven, a place where creativity can be a source of strength and where resilience can be created.

Get ready to be mesmerized by the wonder of ordinary ingredients turned into spectacular food. Allow the recipes on these pages to be your guides as they help you learn the skill of cooking with care and intention. Accept the soothing cadence of dicing, whisking, and boiling, and allow the intricacy of tastes to lead the way.

Within the realm of "Cooking for Comfort and Healing," each meal serves as an act of love, a reminder that despite life's obstacles, there is nourishment, comfort, and healing. I hope this chapter serves as a reminder that cooking is a meaningful way to nourish the spirit and bring comfort and healing to both the cook and the diner. It also provides us with food.

- Recipes tailored for managing chemotherapy side effects

These recipes are designed to address common challenges such as nausea, taste changes, mouth sores, and appetite loss during chemotherapy.

1. **Ginger Lemon Tea:**

- **Ingredients**: Fresh ginger slices, lemon juice, honey, hot water.

- **Preparation:** Steep ginger slices in hot water, add lemon juice and honey. Ginger helps alleviate nausea, while lemon adds flavor.

2. **Banana Oat Smoothie:**

- **Ingredients:** Banana, oats, Greek yogurt, almond milk, honey.

- **Preparation:** Blend banana, oats, yogurt, and almond milk. Honey provides sweetness. Oats soothe the stomach, and banana offers potassium.

3. **Creamy Mashed Potatoes:**

- **Ingredients:** Potatoes, butter, milk, salt, pepper.

- **Preparation:** Boil potatoes, mash with butter and milk. Creamy texture is easy to swallow, and it's gentle on the stomach.

4. **Simple Vegetable Soup:**

- **Ingredients:** Mixed vegetables (carrots, zucchini, spinach), low-sodium broth.

- **Preparation:** Simmer vegetables in broth. Vegetables provide essential nutrients, and the broth keeps it hydrating.

5. **Baked Salmon with Herbs:**

- **Ingredients:** Salmon fillet, olive oil, herbs (rosemary, thyme), lemon.

- **Preparation:** Marinate salmon with herbs and olive oil, bake. Salmon provides omega-3 fatty acids, gentle on the stomach.

6. **Brown Rice Stir-Fry:**

- **Ingredients:** Brown rice, tofu/chicken, mixed vegetables, low-sodium soy sauce.

- **Preparation:** Cook brown rice, stir-fry tofu/chicken and vegetables, add soy sauce. Brown rice offers fiber, and stir-frying makes it easy to digest.

7. **Avocado and Banana Smoothie:**

- **Ingredients:** Avocado, banana, almond milk, honey.

- **Preparation:** Blend avocado, banana, almond milk, and honey. Avocado provides healthy fats and banana adds potassium.

8. **Yogurt Parfait with Berries:**

- **Ingredients:** Greek yogurt, mixed berries, granola, honey.

- **Preparation:** Layer yogurt, berries, and granola. Berries offer antioxidants, and yogurt provides probiotics.

9. **Soothing Chamomile Tea:**

- **Ingredients:** Chamomile tea bags, hot water, honey (optional).

- **Preparation:** Steep chamomile tea bags in hot water, add honey if desired. Chamomile helps with relaxation and digestion.

10. **Lemon Herb Chicken:**

- **Ingredients:** Chicken breast, lemon juice, garlic, herbs (parsley, thyme).

- **Preparation:** Marinate chicken with lemon juice, garlic, and herbs, bake. Lemon adds flavor, and herbs are gentle on the stomach.

11. Quinoa Salad with Feta and Spinach:

- **Ingredients:** Cooked quinoa, fresh spinach, feta cheese, olive oil, lemon juice.

- **Preparation:** Toss quinoa, spinach, and feta. Drizzle with olive oil and lemon juice. Quinoa provides protein, and spinach offers iron.

12. Creamy Pumpkin Soup:

- **Ingredients:** Pumpkin puree, coconut milk, ginger, nutmeg, vegetable broth.

- **Preparation:** Cook pumpkin with ginger and nutmeg, blend with coconut milk and vegetable broth. Pumpkin is easy to digest and comforting.

13. **Mango Banana Smoothie:**

- **Ingredients:** Mango, banana, Greek yogurt, almond milk.

- **Preparation:** Blend mango, banana, yogurt, and almond milk. Mango provides vitamin C, and yogurt adds protein.

14. **Soft Scrambled Eggs:**

- **Ingredients:** Eggs, butter, salt, pepper.

- **Preparation:** Scramble eggs with butter, season with salt and pepper. Soft texture is easy to chew and swallow.

15. **Herbal Infused Water:**

- **Ingredients**: Fresh mint leaves, cucumber slices, lime slices, cold water.

- **Preparation:** Infuse water with mint, cucumber, and lime. Refreshing and hydrating, helps with taste changes.

16. **Miso Soup with Tofu and Seaweed:**

- **Ingredients**: Miso paste, tofu, seaweed, green onions.

- **Preparation:** Dissolve miso paste in hot water, add tofu, seaweed, and green onions. Miso is soothing, and seaweed provides minerals.

17. **Peanut Butter Banana Toast:**

- **Ingredients:** Whole-grain bread, peanut butter, banana slices.

- **Preparation**: Spread peanut butter on toast, top with banana slices. Provides protein, fiber, and potassium.

18. **Honey-Lemon Ginger Water:**

- **Ingredients:** Honey, lemon juice, ginger slices, hot water.

- **Preparation:** Mix honey, lemon juice, and ginger in hot water. Soothes the throat and aids digestion.

19. Cottage Cheese and Pineapple Bowl:

- **Ingredients:** Cottage cheese, fresh pineapple chunks.

- **Preparation:** Combine cottage cheese and pineapple. Cottage cheese offers protein, and pineapple adds a refreshing twist.

20. Steamed Vegetables with Olive Oil and Herbs:

- **Ingredients:** Assorted vegetables (broccoli, carrots, cauliflower), olive oil, herbs (thyme, rosemary).

- **Preparation:** Steam vegetables, drizzle with olive oil and herbs. Retains nutrients and adds flavor without being too heavy.

These recipes are designed to be gentle on the stomach, easy to swallow, and packed with essential nutrients to support the body during chemotherapy. Adjustments can be made based on individual preferences and dietary restrictions, ensuring that each meal is both nourishing and satisfying.

- Delicious and nourishing dishes to soothe the palate

These dishes are not only flavorful but also gentle on the senses, making them perfect choices for individuals experiencing taste changes, nausea, or other side effects.

1. **Creamy Butternut Squash Soup:**

- **Ingredients:** Butternut squash, coconut milk, vegetable broth, ginger, nutmeg.

- **Preparation:** Roast squash, blend with coconut milk, vegetable broth, and spices. Creamy and comforting.

2. **Lemon-Honey Baked Chicken:**

- **Ingredients:** Chicken thighs, lemon juice, honey, garlic, thyme.

- **Preparation:** Marinate chicken with lemon, honey, and herbs, then bake. Sweet and tangy flavors.

3. **Ginger Rice Porridge:**

- **Ingredients:** Rice, ginger, chicken or vegetable broth, green onions.

- **Preparation:** Cook rice with ginger and broth until creamy. Garnish with green onions. Soothing and easy to digest.

4. **Mashed Sweet Potatoes:**

- **Ingredients:** Sweet potatoes, butter, cinnamon, nutmeg.

- **Preparation:** Boil sweet potatoes, mash with butter and spices. Naturally sweet and soft texture.

5. **Soothing Chamomile Panna Cotta:**

- **Ingredients:** Heavy cream, chamomile tea, honey, gelatin.

- **Preparation:** Infuse cream with chamomile, mix with honey and gelatin, then refrigerate. Delicate and calming dessert.

6. **Baked Salmon with Dill Sauce:**

- **Ingredients:** Salmon fillet, yogurt, dill, lemon juice, garlic.

- **Preparation:** Bake salmon, top with yogurt, dill, and lemon-garlic sauce. Fresh and flavorful.

7. **Creamed Spinach:**

- **Ingredients:** Spinach, cream, Parmesan cheese, garlic.

- **Preparation:** Sauté spinach with garlic, mix with cream and cheese. Creamy and nutritious side dish.

8. **Mango-Coconut Chia Pudding:**

- **Ingredients:** Chia seeds, coconut milk, mango puree, honey.

- **Preparation:** Mix chia seeds with coconut milk, layer with mango puree. Sweet, creamy, and packed with nutrients.

9. **Herbal Infused Watermelon Salad:**

- **Ingredients:** Watermelon cubes, mint leaves, feta cheese, balsamic glaze.

- **Preparation:** Toss watermelon with mint, top with crumbled feta, and drizzle with balsamic glaze. Refreshing and hydrating.

10. **Creamy Avocado Pasta:**

- **Ingredients:** Avocado, whole-grain pasta, lemon juice, basil, cherry tomatoes.

- **Preparation:** Blend avocado, lemon juice, and basil, toss with cooked pasta and cherry tomatoes. Creamy and light.

11. Ginger-Lemon Herbal Tea:

- **Ingredients:** Fresh ginger slices, lemon zest, honey, hot water.

- **Preparation:** Steep ginger and lemon zest in hot water, add honey. A soothing drink for relaxation.

12. Roasted Vegetable Medley:

- **Ingredients:** Assorted vegetables (carrots, bell peppers, zucchini), olive oil, herbs.

- **Preparation:** Roast vegetables with olive oil and herbs. Tender and flavorful side dish.

13. Cucumber and Mint Yogurt Dip:

- **Ingredients:** Greek yogurt, cucumber, mint, garlic, lemon juice.

- **Preparation:** Grate cucumber, mix with yogurt, mint, garlic, and lemon juice. Cooling and refreshing dip.

14. **Pumpkin Seed Trail Mix:**

- **Ingredients:** Pumpkin seeds, almonds, dried cranberries, dark chocolate chips.

- **Preparation:** Mix seeds, nuts, cranberries, and chocolate chips. A crunchy, nutrient-packed snack.

15. **Herbal Infused Roasted Chicken:**

- **Ingredients:** Chicken breast, rosemary, thyme, sage, garlic.

- **Preparation:** Marinate chicken with herbs and garlic, then roast. Fragrant and flavorful.

16. **Lavender-Infused Honey:**

- **Ingredients:** Lavender buds, honey.

- **Preparation:** Infuse lavender buds in honey for a few days. Drizzle over desserts or in herbal tea for a soothing touch.

17. **Creamy Coconut Rice Pudding:**

- **Ingredients:** Arborio rice, coconut milk, sugar, vanilla extract.

- **Preparation:** Cook rice with coconut milk, sugar, and vanilla until creamy. Comforting dessert.

18. **Peppermint Chocolate Smoothie:**

- **Ingredients:** Banana, almond milk, cocoa powder, peppermint extract.

- **Preparation:** Blend banana, almond milk, cocoa powder, and a few drops of peppermint extract. Refreshing and indulgent.

19. **Baked Apples with Cinnamon:**

- **Ingredients:** Apples, cinnamon, nutmeg, honey.

- **Preparation:** Core apples, sprinkle with cinnamon and nutmeg, drizzle with honey, then bake. Warm and comforting dessert.

20. **Ginger-Lemon Sorbet:**

- **Ingredients:** Fresh ginger, lemon juice, sugar, water.

- **Preparation:** Make a ginger-lemon syrup, freeze, then

- Easy-to-follow meal preparation tips and techniques

Every kitchen has a sanctuary at its center, where comforting fragrances waft through the air and ingredients combine to create elixirs of healing. Welcome to the magical chapter "Cooking for Comfort and Healing," where delicate caregiving blends with culinary expertise. Here, amid the sounds of pans sizzling and spices wafting, you'll set off on a journey that goes beyond simple sustenance to replenish the soul.

When things are tough and you feel vulnerable, there is great comfort in cooking. It's a ritual, an intimate dance between the hands that prepare and the hearts that seek comfort, rather than just a simple melding of flavors and textures. This chapter honors the ability of food to serve as more than just a source of nourishment; it may also act as a source of warmth, a spiritual healer, and a ray of hope.

Imagine the rich aroma of a pot of soup simmering on the stove or the soft kneading of bread by skilled hands. These are not only culinary pursuits; they are acts of love, infused with the deep knowledge that feeding transcends the material world. It reaches the very center of who we are, providing nourishment for both our tired bodies and souls.

You will find a plethora of recipes in the pages that follow, all of which have been painstakingly prepared and selected for their capacity to soothe and heal. Every meal is a testament to the soothing power of mindful cooking, from delicately flavored teas that calm the senses to velvety soups that embrace like a warm embrace. You will learn from these recipes that the kitchen can serve as a haven, a place where creativity can be a source of strength and where resilience can be created.

Get ready to be mesmerized by the wonder of ordinary ingredients turned into spectacular food. Allow the recipes on these pages to be your guides as they help you learn the skill of cooking with care and intention. Accept the soothing cadence of dicing, whisking, and boiling, and allow the intricacy of tastes to lead the way.

Within the realm of "Cooking for Comfort and Healing," each meal serves as an act of love, a reminder that despite life's obstacles, there is nourishment, comfort, and healing. I hope this chapter serves as a reminder that cooking is a meaningful way to nourish the spirit and bring comfort and healing to both the cook and the diner. It also provides us with food.

1. **Carefully Follow Recipes:**

Pro tip: Before you begin cooking, go over the entire recipe. Recognize the procedures and get all the ingredients ready in advance.

Example: Following the instructions exactly guarantees that every layer of a complicated dish like lasagna is put together correctly and tastes well.

2. **Harmonize Flavors:**

Advice: Recognize how to harmonize sweet, salty, sour, and savory flavors. As you cook, taste and adjust the seasonings.

Example: To create a well-rounded flavor profile in a stir-fry, balance the sweetness of hoisin sauce with the saltiness of soy sauce and the freshness of lime juice.

3. **Try New Herbs and Spices:**

Tip: Experiment with various herbs and spices to improve the flavor of your food. Try out different flavors without fear.

Example: To enhance the flavor of roasted vegetables, add cumin and paprika to the sauce, or add herbs like basil and oregano to pasta sauces.

4. **Develop Time Management Skills:**

Advice: Master multitasking and effective time management in the kitchen. Tasks requiring longer cooking times should be started first.

Example: Prepare salad items or marinate proteins for a later dinner while the boiling of a soup.

5. **Maintain Organization While Cooking:**

Advice: Keep your work area tidy and orderly. To

prevent clutter, keep ingredients and garbage in different containers.

Example: To make it easy to add premeasured ingredients to your recipes without fumbling with containers, place them in small bowls or ramekins.

6. **Work on Timing and Patience**: A helpful hint is to be patient, particularly when baking or simmering. Cook your meal according to the recommended timings and try not to check on it too much.

For instance, to ensure consistent and fluffy results when baking a cake, try not to open the oven door too often.

7. **Accept Batch Cooking:**

Advice: Make big quantities of basic foods like grains, beans, or sauces and freeze them in portion-sized freezer bags for quick and simple meals later on.

Example: Prepare a large quantity of quinoa and portion it out into freezer-safe bags. As required, thaw and reheat different dishes.

8. **Cook with Mindfulness:**

Pro Tip: When cooking, stay in the present. To improve your cooking, pay attention to flavors, textures, and scents.

Example: To ensure a rich flavor without bitterness, when sautéing garlic, pay attention to the aroma and regulate the heat to avoid it from burning.

9. **Clean while You Go:** Here's a tip to keep your workspace clutter-free and simplify cleanup after meals: wash dishes and utensils while you cook.

Example: To keep your workplace tidy, wash the cutting board and knife you used to chop the vegetables while your soup is boiling.

Meal preparation becomes more efficient, pleasurable, and fulfilling when you incorporate these simple meal preparation tips and strategies into your daily routine. Cheers to cooking!

CHAPTER 4: NUTRIENT-PACKED RECIPE COLLECTION

Welcome to a gastronomic trip that goes beyond the typical and explores the worlds of nourishment and enjoyment! This chapter is filled with an abundance of flavors, colors, and scents that have been thoughtfully chosen to stimulate your senses and entice your palate. This is more than simply a list of recipes; it's a symphony of nutrient-dense treats, with each recipe painstakingly prepared to provide your body energy, harmony, and unadulterated goodness.

Within the domain of the Nutrient-Packed Recipe Collection, each recipe narrates a tale of healthful components coming together harmoniously, led by the mastery of culinary skills and a profound comprehension of nutritional science. These foods are more than just a gastronomic feast; they are a celebration of the richness that nature offers, cooked into mouthwatering creations that uplift the spirit and the body.

Imagine the colors of crisp veggies, the searing of meats over a hot grill, and the aroma of herbs bringing their flavor to simmering sauces. Every dish is evidence of the conviction that food is a source of life, vitality, and deep happiness in addition to being a means of subsistence. This selection has been thoughtfully chosen to satisfy every craving and gastronomic curiosity, whether you're looking for the cozy comforts of home-cooked classics, the exotic attraction of international cuisine, or the creative fusion of flavors.

Be ready to go on a hunt for the ideal ratio of flavor to nutrition as you set out on this culinary adventure. Each dish is created with your health in mind and is packed with ingredients that are high in vitamins, minerals, antioxidants, and other vital nutrients. These recipes show how luxury and health can live in harmony on your plate and are more than just meals—they are a monument to the transformational power of a balanced diet.

These pages contain more than simply recipes; they also serve as a source of creativity for preparing colorful, healthful meals that capture the spirit of a well-fed existence. Put on your apron, polish your knives, and get set to discover a world in which every mouthful is a celebration, every taste a revelation, and every dinner a declaration of your dedication to overall well-being. Greetings and welcome to the Nutrient-Packed Recipe Collection, a taste sensation that will satiate your need for more bite after delicious bite.

- A diverse array of recipes featuring cancer-fighting ingredients

A diverse array of recipes featuring cancer-fighting ingredients is not only a delightful culinary experience but also a proactive step toward promoting overall health and well-being. In this section, we will explore a variety of recipes, each carefully crafted with ingredients known for their cancer-fighting properties, accompanied by relevant examples and explanations:

1. **Grilled Salmon with Turmeric and Lemon:**

- **Ingredients**: Salmon fillet, turmeric powder, lemon juice, garlic, olive oil.

- **Explanation**: Salmon is rich in omega-3 fatty acids, while turmeric contains curcumin, known for its anti-inflammatory properties. Combined with the freshness of lemon, this dish provides a burst of flavors and health benefits.

2. **Kale and Berry Salad with Walnuts:**

- **Ingredients:** Kale, mixed berries (blueberries, strawberries), walnuts, feta cheese, balsamic vinaigrette.

- **Explanation:** Kale is a cruciferous vegetable containing sulforaphane, a compound with potential cancer-fighting properties. Berries are packed with antioxidants, and walnuts provide healthy fats and protein, creating a vibrant and nutritious salad.

3. **Quinoa and Vegetable Stir-Fry:**

- **Ingredients:** Quinoa, broccoli, bell peppers, carrots, tofu (optional), soy sauce.

- **Explanation:** Quinoa is a whole grain rich in fiber and nutrients. Broccoli, bell peppers, and carrots are high in vitamins and antioxidants. Tofu adds plant-based protein, making this stir-fry a balanced and wholesome choice.

4. **Tomato and Basil Whole Wheat Pasta:**

- **Ingredients:** Whole wheat pasta, fresh tomatoes, garlic, basil, olive oil, Parmesan cheese.

- **Explanation:** Tomatoes are a great source of lycopene, a powerful antioxidant. Basil contains compounds like flavonoids, which have potential cancer-fighting properties. Whole wheat pasta provides fiber and nutrients, making it a hearty and healthful dish.

5. **Chickpea and Spinach Curry:**

- **Ingredients:** Chickpeas, spinach, tomatoes, onions, garlic, ginger, curry spices.

- **Explanation:** Chickpeas are rich in fiber and protein. Spinach contains various vitamins and minerals. The combination of these ingredients with aromatic spices creates a flavorful and nourishing curry.

6. **Citrus and Avocado Salad:**

- **Ingredients**: Mixed greens, oranges, grapefruit, avocado, almonds, citrus vinaigrette.

- **Explanation:** Citrus fruits like oranges and grapefruit are high in vitamin C and antioxidants. Avocado provides healthy fats, and almonds add a crunchy texture. This refreshing salad is both tangy and satisfying.

7. Green Tea Infused Poached Chicken:

- **Ingredients:** Chicken breast, green tea bags, ginger, garlic, scallions.

- **Explanation:** Green tea is rich in antioxidants, especially catechins. Poaching chicken in green tea enhances its flavor and infuses it with the health benefits of tea, creating a light and aromatic dish.

8. Berry and Yogurt Parfait:

- **Ingredients:** Greek yogurt, mixed berries (strawberries, raspberries), honey, granola.

- **Explanation:** Greek yogurt is high in protein and probiotics. Berries provide vitamins and antioxidants. Honey adds natural sweetness, and granola provides crunch. Layering these ingredients creates a delicious and nutritious dessert or breakfast option.

9. **Roasted Turmeric Cauliflower:**

   - **Ingredients:** Cauliflower florets, turmeric powder, cumin, coriander, olive oil.

   - **Explanation:** Cauliflower is a cruciferous vegetable with potential cancer-fighting properties. Turmeric's active compound, curcumin, has anti-inflammatory and antioxidant effects. Roasting cauliflower with these spices results in a flavorful and healthful side dish.

10. **Sweet Potato and Black Bean Tacos:**

   - **Ingredients:** Sweet potato, black beans, corn tortillas, avocado, salsa, cilantro.

   - **Explanation:** Sweet potatoes are rich in beta-carotene, while black beans provide fiber and protein. Avocado adds creaminess and healthy fats. Combining these ingredients in tacos offers a satisfying and nutritious meal option.

These diverse and delectable recipes showcase the versatility of cancer-fighting ingredients. By incorporating these dishes into your diet, you not only indulge in culinary delights but also take proactive steps toward supporting your health and well-being. Embrace the flavors, savor the nutrients, and enjoy the journey to a healthier you through the power of nourishing foods.

- *Breakfast, lunch, dinner, and snack options for different dietary requirements*

Here's a breakdown of breakfast, lunch, dinner, and snack options tailored for various dietary requirements, all featuring cancer-fighting ingredients. Each meal option is designed to accommodate specific dietary needs while incorporating nutritious and flavorful ingredients known for their potential cancer-fighting properties:

Breakfast:

1. **Gluten-Free Breakfast Bowl:**

- **Ingredients:** Quinoa, mixed berries (blueberries, raspberries), almonds, chia seeds, honey.

- **Explanation:** Quinoa provides protein and fiber. Berries offer antioxidants, while almonds add healthy fats. Chia seeds are rich in omega-3 fatty acids. Drizzle with honey for natural sweetness.

2. **Vegan Smoothie Bowl:**

- **Ingredients:** Spinach, banana, almond milk, flaxseeds, kiwi, and coconut flakes.

- **Explanation:** Spinach is a leafy green rich in vitamins and minerals. Almond milk is a dairy-free alternative. Flaxseeds provide omega-3 fatty acids. Kiwi adds vitamin C. Garnish with coconut flakes for texture.

Lunch:

1. **Paleo Grilled Chicken Salad:**

- **Ingredients:** Grilled chicken breast, mixed greens, avocado, cherry tomatoes, pumpkin seeds, olive oil, lemon juice.

- **Explanation:** Grilled chicken offers lean protein. Avocado provides healthy fats. Pumpkin seeds contain antioxidants. Olive oil and lemon juice make a light dressing.

2. **Keto Zucchini Noodles with Pesto:**

- **Ingredients:** Zucchini noodles, pesto sauce (basil, garlic, pine nuts, olive oil), cherry tomatoes, Parmesan cheese.

- **Explanation:** Zucchini noodles are low in carbs. Pesto contains basil, a herb with potential cancer-fighting compounds. Tomatoes offer lycopene. Garnish with Parmesan cheese.

Dinner:

1. **Mediterranean Baked Salmon:**

- **Ingredients:** Salmon fillet, olives, tomatoes, artichokes, garlic, olive oil, lemon, fresh herbs (rosemary, thyme).

- **Explanation:** Salmon is rich in omega-3 fatty acids. Olives and olive oil provide monounsaturated fats. Tomatoes contain lycopene. Artichokes offer dietary fiber and antioxidants.

2. **Vegetarian Stir-Fry with Tofu:**

- **Ingredients:** Tofu, broccoli, bell peppers, carrots, snow peas, soy sauce, ginger, garlic.

- **Explanation:** Tofu is a plant-based protein source. Broccoli and bell peppers are high in vitamins and antioxidants. Ginger and garlic have anti-inflammatory properties.

Snacks:

1. **Nuts and Seeds Trail Mix:**

- **Ingredients:** Almonds, walnuts, pumpkin seeds, dried cranberries.

- **Explanation:** Almonds and walnuts offer healthy fats and antioxidants. Pumpkin seeds provide fiber and minerals. Cranberries add a touch of sweetness.

2. **Greek Yogurt Parfait with Berries:**

- **Ingredients:** Greek yogurt, mixed berries (strawberries, blueberries), honey, granola.

- **Explanation:** Greek yogurt is high in protein and probiotics. Berries offer vitamins and antioxidants. Honey provides natural sweetness. Granola adds crunch.

By tailoring these meal options to different dietary requirements, individuals can enjoy a variety of delicious and cancer-fighting dishes while adhering to their specific needs. Whether following a gluten-free, vegan, paleo, keto, or vegetarian diet, these meals and snacks showcase the versatility of cancer-fighting ingredients and promote overall well-being.

- Culinary inspiration for every stage of chemotherapy

Navigating the challenges of chemotherapy can be daunting, but the power of culinary inspiration can play a significant role in supporting patients through every stage of their journey. From combatting taste changes to boosting energy levels, here are personalized culinary ideas for each stage of chemotherapy, each featuring relevant examples:

1. **Pre-Chemotherapy Preparation:**

Cancer-Fighting Smoothie Preparations:

- **Ingredients:** Spinach, kale, berries (blueberries, raspberries), banana, Greek yogurt, almond milk.

- **Explanation:** Blend leafy greens with antioxidant-rich berries, banana for natural sweetness, and protein-packed Greek yogurt. Freeze in portions for easy access when energy levels are low.

Meal Prepping Hearty Soups:

- **Ingredients:** Lentils, carrots, tomatoes, garlic, turmeric, ginger.

- **Explanation:** Prepare lentil-based soups with immune-boosting turmeric and ginger. Freeze in batches for quick and nourishing meals before and after chemotherapy sessions.

2. **During Chemotherapy Treatments:**

Gentle and Hydrating Infusions:

- **Ingredients:** Fresh mint leaves, cucumber slices, lemon slices, cold water.

- **Explanation:** Infuse water with mint, cucumber, and lemon for a refreshing, hydrating drink during treatments, helping combat nausea and keeping the body hydrated.

Comforting Rice Congee:

- **Ingredients:** Rice, chicken or vegetable broth, shredded chicken (optional), green onions.

- **Explanation:** Cook rice in a broth until it reaches a porridge-like consistency. Add shredded chicken if desired, garnish with green onions. Easy to digest and soothing for the stomach.

3. Post-Chemotherapy Recovery:

Protein-Packed Recovery Smoothies:

- **Ingredients:** Greek yogurt, banana, peanut butter, honey, almond milk.

- **Explanation:** Blend Greek yogurt with banana, peanut butter for protein, and a drizzle of honey for sweetness. This smoothie provides essential nutrients for recovery.

Nutrient-Dense Buddha Bowls:

- **Ingredients:** Quinoa, roasted vegetables (sweet potatoes, broccoli, bell peppers), avocado slices, tahini sauce.

- **Explanation:** Assemble a Buddha bowl with quinoa, roasted vegetables, creamy avocado, and drizzle with tahini sauce. Packed with vitamins, minerals, and healthy fats for post-chemotherapy recovery.

4. Long-Term Recovery and Well-being:

Anti-Inflammatory Turmeric Curry:

- **Ingredients**: Turmeric, chickpeas, spinach, tomatoes, onions, garlic, coconut milk.

- **Explanation:** Prepare a curry with turmeric, chickpeas, and vegetables. Turmeric's curcumin has anti-inflammatory properties, aiding in long-term recovery and overall well-being.

Green Tea Infused Desserts:

- **Ingredients:** Green tea powder, Greek yogurt, honey, fresh berries.

- **Explanation:** Incorporate antioxidant-rich green tea powder into desserts like Greek yogurt parfaits. Top with honey and fresh berries for a delightful treat that supports overall health.

Each of these culinary ideas is tailored to specific stages of chemotherapy, offering not just nourishment but also comfort, taste, and variety. By embracing these creative recipes, patients can find inspiration in their meals, making the culinary aspect of their journey a source of support and positivity during every step of their chemotherapy experience.

CHAPTER 5: SUSTAINING WELLNESS BEYOND TREATMENT

Welcome to the empowering chapter, where the journey becomes a beautiful tapestry of prolonged well-being, resilience, and renewed strength, rather than ending with the final treatment. We take a deep dive into life after the storm in "Sustaining Wellness beyond Treatment," where we embrace health, happiness, and a fresh lease on life. This chapter is more than just a list of recommendations; it's a ray of hope, a guide for facing the future with unflinching energy and optimism.

Imagine living in a place where each morning holds the possibility of healing, where every meal is an occasion to celebrate life, and where hope permeates every second of every day. Here, we go deeply into the practice of thriving after treatment—rather than merely getting by. Armed with information, resiliency, and a profound comprehension of the body's extraordinary capacity for healing and rejuvenation, we bravely traverse the ocean of uncertainty.

"Sustaining Wellness beyond Treatment" is not just a manual; rather, it is a monument to the extraordinary power that is already within you and just needs to be let loose. We reveal the keys to maintaining your physical, emotional, and mental well-being in this chapter, giving you priceless knowledge, useful advice, and sincere inspiration to live life to the fullest.

We'll delve into the benefits of healing foods, mind-body techniques, restorative workouts, and the transformational potential of self-care. This chapter is full of inspiration, lighting the sparks of optimism and self-love that drive the path to long-lasting wellness, from practicing mindfulness to creating meaningful connections and rekindling passions.

However, this chapter is about more than just you; it's about the network of people who have travelled similar routes, the loved ones who support you, and the community of support that is all around you. It's an observance of the unity, kindness, and steadfast spirit that characterize the human condition.

You may expect to be inspired, motivated, and profoundly moved as you flip the pages. Allow this chapter to be your constant support system as you embrace the countless opportunities that life after treatment has to offer. It can also serve as your guide. Together, we set out on a life-changing journey that surpasses the difficulties of the past and opens up a future of unending happiness, health, and opportunity. Greetings from the journey of maintaining well-being after treatment. The journey starts over.

- Strategies for transitioning to a post-chemotherapy diet

Transitioning to a post-chemotherapy diet is a significant step toward reclaiming your health and well-being. It involves careful consideration of your body's needs and making conscious choices to support your recovery. Here are strategies, each accompanied by relevant examples, to guide you through this crucial transition:

1. **Gradual Reintroduction of Foods:**

   - **Strategy:** Gradually reintroduce foods that were restricted during chemotherapy, such as raw fruits and vegetables, to allow your digestive system to adjust.

   - **Example:** Start with easily digestible cooked vegetables like steamed carrots and gradually incorporate raw salads with mixed greens, tomatoes, and cucumbers.

2. **Focus on Whole, Nutrient-Dense Foods:**

- **Strategy:** Prioritize whole foods rich in nutrients, vitamins, and minerals to support overall health and boost your immune system.

- **Example:** Include foods like quinoa, lean proteins (chicken, fish, tofu), colorful fruits and vegetables, whole grains, and healthy fats (avocado, nuts) in your daily meals.

3. **Embrace Anti-Inflammatory Foods:**

- **Strategy:** Choose foods with anti-inflammatory properties to reduce inflammation and promote healing in your body.

- **Example:** Incorporate turmeric into curries, drink green tea for its antioxidant content, and consume fatty fish like salmon, rich in omega-3 fatty acids.

4. **Stay Hydrated:**

- **Strategy:** Drink plenty of water and consume hydrating foods to stay well-hydrated, especially if you experience lingering effects like dry mouth or altered taste.

- **Example:** Infuse your water with slices of cucumber, lemon, and mint for a refreshing twist, and consume water-rich foods like watermelon and oranges.

5. **Monitor Portion Sizes:**

- Strategy: Be mindful of portion sizes to avoid overeating and support a healthy weight, which is important for overall well-being.

- **Example:** Use smaller plates to control portions and focus on balanced meals with appropriate servings of proteins, carbohydrates, and vegetables.

6. **Include Probiotic-Rich Foods:**

- Strategy: Integrate probiotic-rich foods to promote gut health, aid digestion, and enhance your immune system.

- Example: Incorporate yogurt with live cultures, kefir, sauerkraut, and kimchi into your diet for natural probiotic sources.

7. Listen to Your Body:

- Strategy: Pay attention to how your body responds to different foods. Note any sensitivities or allergies and adjust your diet accordingly.

- Example: If dairy products cause discomfort, opt for lactose-free alternatives like almond milk or lactose-free yogurt.

8. Seek Professional Guidance:

- Strategy: Consult a registered dietitian or nutritionist experienced in post-chemotherapy diets to create a personalized meal plan tailored to your specific needs.

- **Example:** Work with a professional to create a customized meal plan that aligns with your dietary preferences, restrictions, and health goals.

9. **Practice Mindful Eating:**

- **Strategy:** Practice mindful eating to savor each bite, improve digestion, and enhance your overall relationship with food.

- **Example:** Engage your senses by appreciating the colors, textures, and flavors of your meals. Chew slowly and be present in the moment.

10. **Include Adaptogenic Herbs:**

- **Strategy:** Integrate adaptogenic herbs like ashwagandha and holy basil to support your body's stress response and promote overall resilience.

- **Example:** Brew herbal teas with adaptogenic herbs or add powdered forms to smoothies for their potential health benefits.

By incorporating these strategies and examples into your post-chemotherapy diet, you're not just nourishing your body; you're also fostering a sense of empowerment and well-being. Remember that this transition is unique to you, and it's essential to be patient and compassionate with yourself throughout this process. Celebrate each step forward, embrace the healing power of nutritious foods, and revel in the renewed vitality that a well-balanced diet can bring to your life.

- Long-term dietary recommendations for cancer survivors

Long-term dietary recommendations for cancer survivors are essential for maintaining overall health, supporting the body's recovery, and reducing the risk of cancer recurrence. These recommendations focus on promoting a balanced, nutrient-rich diet that supports the immune system, provides energy, and aids in the prevention of other chronic illnesses. Here are strategies, each accompanied by relevant examples, to guide cancer survivors towards a healthy and fulfilling long-term dietary plan:

1. **Prioritize Plant-Based Foods:**

 - **Strategy:** Emphasize a variety of fruits, vegetables, whole grains, legumes, and nuts. Plant-based foods are rich in vitamins, minerals, antioxidants, and fiber, promoting overall health.

 - **Examples:** Include colorful vegetables like spinach, kale, and carrots; whole grains like brown rice and quinoa; fruits such as berries, oranges, and apples; and protein sources like lentils, chickpeas, and almonds.

2. **Choose Lean Proteins:**

 - **Strategy:** Opt for lean protein sources such as poultry, fish, tofu, legumes, and low-fat dairy.

Lean proteins aid in muscle repair and immune function without adding excessive saturated fats.

- **Examples:** Include grilled chicken breast, salmon, tofu stir-fry, lentil soup, and low-fat yogurt in your meals.

3. **Limit Processed Foods and Sugars:**

- **Strategy:** Reduce intake of processed foods, sugary snacks, and sugary beverages. These items can contribute to inflammation and negatively impact overall health.

- **Examples:** Avoid sugary sodas and candies; opt for fresh fruit instead of sugary desserts; choose whole grains over sugary cereals.

4. **Incorporate Healthy Fats:**

- **Strategy:** Include sources of healthy fats like avocados, nuts, seeds, and olive oil. Healthy fats are essential for brain health and the absorption of certain vitamins.

- **Examples:** Use olive oil for salad dressings, snack on a handful of mixed nuts, spread avocado on whole-grain toast, and sprinkle chia seeds on yogurt.

5. **Stay Hydrated:**

- **Strategy:** Drink plenty of water throughout the day to stay well-hydrated. Proper hydration supports digestion, circulation, and overall bodily functions.

- **Examples:** Besides water, consume hydrating foods like watermelon, cucumbers, oranges, and herbal teas.

6. **Practice Portion Control:**

- **Strategy:** Be mindful of portion sizes to maintain a healthy weight and prevent overeating. Portion control is crucial for managing calorie intake.

- **Examples:** Use smaller plates, listen to your body's hunger and fullness cues, and avoid second servings if you're not genuinely hungry.

7. Include Foods Rich in Antioxidants:

- **Strategy:** Antioxidants help combat free radicals in the body, reducing the risk of chronic diseases. Include foods rich in antioxidants such as berries, leafy greens, and colorful vegetables.

- **Examples:** Consume blueberries in your breakfast, add spinach to salads, and snack on antioxidant-rich dark chocolate (in moderation).

8. Moderate Alcohol Consumption:

- **Strategy:** If you choose to drink alcohol, do so in moderation. Excessive alcohol consumption is linked to various health issues, including an increased risk of certain cancers.

- **Examples:** Limit alcohol intake to one drink per day for women and two drinks per day for men. One drink is equivalent to 5 ounces of wine,

12 ounces of beer, or 1.5 ounces of distilled spirits.

9. Plan Balanced Meals:

- **Strategy:** Create balanced meals that incorporate a variety of food groups. Balance carbohydrates, proteins, and fats to provide sustained energy and overall nutrition.

- **Examples:** Plan meals like grilled salmon with quinoa and steamed vegetables, or a balanced salad with mixed greens, grilled chicken, nuts, and a variety of colorful vegetables.

10. Maintain Regular Physical Activity:

- **Strategy:** Combine a healthy diet with regular physical activity. Exercise supports overall health, boosts energy levels, and helps maintain a healthy weight.

- **Examples:** Engage in activities you enjoy, such as walking, swimming, yoga, or dancing, for at least 150 minutes of moderate-intensity exercise per week.

By incorporating these strategies and examples into their daily lives, cancer survivors can promote their overall well-being, reduce the risk of cancer recurrence, and embrace a vibrant, healthy lifestyle in the long term. Remember that these recommendations are general guidelines; it's crucial to consult with healthcare providers or registered dietitians to create a personalized dietary plan based on individual health needs and preferences.

- A roadmap for maintaining a health-conscious lifestyle after treatment

Navigating life after cancer treatment requires a thoughtful and health-conscious approach. Establishing a roadmap for this journey involves incorporating positive lifestyle changes that promote well-being and reduce the risk of recurrence. Here's a comprehensive guide, complete with relevant examples, to help maintain a health-conscious lifestyle after treatment:

1. **Embrace Regular Physical Activity:**

   - **Strategy:** Engage in regular exercise to boost energy levels, enhance mood, and improve overall fitness. Aim for a combination of aerobic exercises, strength training, and flexibility exercises.

   - **Examples:** Take daily walks in nature, attend yoga classes for flexibility, do bodyweight exercises at home, or participate in group fitness activities like dance or cycling.

2. **Prioritize Stress Management:**

   - **Strategy:** Practice stress-reducing activities such as meditation, deep breathing exercises, mindfulness, or hobbies to manage stress effectively.

95 |CANCER-FIGHTING CUISINE

- **Examples:** Practice mindfulness meditation for 10 minutes daily, indulge in creative hobbies like painting or gardening, or unwind with a warm bath and calming music.

3. **Adopt a Nutrient-Dense Diet:**

- **Strategy:** Focus on whole foods, lean proteins, fruits, vegetables, and whole grains. Minimize processed foods, sugary snacks, and excessive saturated fats.

- **Examples:** Prepare colorful salads with a variety of vegetables, incorporate lean proteins like grilled chicken or fish, snack on fresh fruits and nuts, and choose whole grains like brown rice or quinoa.

4. **Prioritize Mental Health:**

- **Strategy:** Seek support from mental health professionals if needed. Prioritize activities that bring joy and relaxation, and surround yourself with supportive and positive individuals.

- **Examples:** Engage in therapy or counseling if helpful, spend quality time with loved ones, practice gratitude journaling, and participate in support groups or community activities.

5. Ensure Regular Health Check-ups:

- **Strategy:** Schedule regular follow-up appointments with healthcare providers, including oncologists and primary care physicians, to monitor your health and address any concerns promptly.

- **Examples:** Keep track of follow-up appointments, blood tests, and imaging scans. Discuss any new symptoms or concerns with your healthcare team.

6. Maintain a Healthy Weight:

- **Strategy:** Aim for a healthy weight by balancing your diet with regular exercise. Achieving and maintaining a healthy weight is essential for overall health and well-being.

- **Examples:** Use portion control, incorporate more plant-based foods, and stay active to maintain a healthy weight. Seek guidance from a registered dietitian if necessary.

7. **Stay Hydrated:**

- **Strategy:** Drink an adequate amount of water throughout the day to stay hydrated. Proper hydration supports various bodily functions and overall health.

- **Examples:** Carry a reusable water bottle, set reminders to drink water, and consume hydrating foods like watermelon, cucumbers, and oranges.

8. **Avoid Tobacco and Limit Alcohol:**

- **Strategy:** Avoid tobacco products completely. Limit alcohol consumption to moderate levels, if at all, as excessive alcohol intake is linked to an increased risk of certain cancers.

- **Examples:** Seek support to quit smoking if you are a smoker. Limit alcohol intake to one drink per day for women and two drinks per day for men, if alcohol is consumed.

9. **Cultivate Healthy Sleep Patterns:**

- **Strategy:** Prioritize sleep and establish a consistent sleep routine. Quality sleep is vital for immune function, mood, and overall health.

- **Examples:** Create a relaxing bedtime routine, keep the bedroom cool and dark, limit screen time before sleep, and aim for 7-9 hours of sleep each night.

10. **Engage in Lifelong Learning:**

- **Strategy:** Pursue interests, hobbies, or educational activities that promote mental stimulation and personal growth. Continuous learning fosters a sense of purpose and fulfillment.

- **Examples:** Enroll in online courses, attend workshops or seminars, join book clubs, or engage in creative pursuits like writing, painting, or learning musical instruments.

By following this roadmap and incorporating these health-conscious strategies and examples into your daily life, you can actively contribute to your overall well-being, enhance your quality of life, and reduce the risk of cancer recurrence. Remember that this journey is unique to you, so adapt these strategies to fit your individual preferences and needs. Seek support from healthcare professionals, friends, and family to make this post-treatment phase a fulfilling and empowering experience.

CONCLUSION

As we come to the end of the chapters in "Cancer-Fighting Cuisine: Nutrient-Packed Recipes and Guidance for Every Stage of Chemotherapy," we set out on a journey of empowerment, driven by knowledge, fortitude, and the transforming potential of wholesome foods. We have examined the complex relationship between nutrition and healing through this culinary voyage, tying together the threads of delectable recipes, evidence-based advice, and steadfast support for each stage of chemotherapy.

Let us take the lessons we have learnt from these pages with us as we say our goodbyes. Allow the scents of hearty soups, the vivid hues of salads high in antioxidants, and the satisfying sizzle of nutrient-dense stir fries to linger in your kitchen as a constant reminder of the significant benefits of mindful eating. I hope that the information you have learned about cancer-preventing foods, well-balanced diets, and customized meal plans will enable you to make wise decisions and promote the peaceful coexistence of indulgence and health on your plate.

We have accepted the difficulties that come with chemotherapy in a spirit of harmony, commemorating each stage's victory with delicious meals that feed the body and the soul.

Recall that this book is more than simply a compilation of recipes; it is an ode to your inner strength and a reminder that recovering from illness can be a delicious and uplifting experience.

May you find comfort in the kitchen, happiness in every bite, and the awareness that you are the key to your well-being as you travel on after reading these pages? Every nutrient-dense meal you cook is an opportunity to nourish your body, uplift your soul, and greet life with renewed vigor.

Cheers to your enduring well-being, an exciting future, and an infinite amount of opportunities for your culinary pursuits. I hope that you have excellent health, delectable tastes, and a steadfast faith in the curative properties of cancer-fighting cuisine.

9 798867 082727